THE STYLE CHALLENGE

A 9-step guide to creating a capsule wardrobe and a curated closet you will love

A. EDMOND

The Style Challenge by A. Edmond

Published by A. Edmond

340 S Lemon Ave #8227, Walnut CA 91789 USA

www.minimalism.co

info@minimalism.co

Cover by A. Edmond

First Edition

Contents

Invitation

Welcome style enthusiasts. The Style Challenge is a lightweight manual designed to help you curate your closet and create a simple, signature style. However, it is just the start of your personal style journey and overall exploration of self-image.

I invite you to join my personal growth platform that is dedicated to empowering you with simple strategies that streamline your life. As a personal growth coach, business consultant and creative entrepreneur my work reaches over 1 million like-minded individuals and I'd be thrilled if you joined the community.

Start by downloading the companion guide to The Style Challenge at **minimalism.co/style** which will help you complete the enclosed exercises, and I'll send you a wealth of additional personal growth resources to further support you.

Introduction

Only great minds can afford a simple style — Stendhal

The Style Challenge is the third book in my Streamline Your Life series that empowers you with simple strategies to improve your life.

Several years ago I sold or gave away about 90% of my possessions. I was going through a number of exciting life changes (new country, new career, and so on) in that period and I used that momentum to more fully realize my minimalistic ideals. Since then I've continued to experience a lot of change and, as a result, I've only been able to hold onto a few possessions.

I'm sure you know that change isn't always easy. Living a long time without certain things that genuinely enhance your sense of self sounds admirable but it's not comfortable. So, I turned my attention to wardrobe and thought about how I could create a signature style from only a few pieces. I came up with a 9-step process that included:

1. Match your wardrobe to your lifestyle

2. Develop a distinct aesthetic

3. Evaluate what should stay or go

4. Create a shopping checklist

5. Budget for any wardrobe needs

6. Determine a set of "go-to" brands

7. Shop without impulse purchasing

8. Increase the longevity of your clothing

   Maintain your commitment to a simple style

A simple style constitutes a well-curated closet made up of intentional purchases of essential items that compliment your shape, aesthetic, and lifestyle. It's the outcome of thoughtfully selecting pieces with the perfect fit, fabrics, and colors for you.

Can you imagine every item you own being something that looks great on you and that you absolutely love to wear? Well, that's exactly what I want to help you accomplish.

So many smart and successful people – from Albert Einstein and Steve Jobs to Former President Barack Obama and Drew Barrymore – have opted for a pared down and highly streamlined wardrobe. In fact, you may already be familiar with trendy, simple style concepts such as the "Capsule Wardrobe" and "Daily Uniform".

Why is a simple style increasingly becoming such a popular way to dress? It's because it eases decision-making, allowing you to more efficiently allocate your precious resources (time, energy, money) to more pressing matters. It also gives you a sense of continuity and, thus, confidence in your own signature style.

In this book we are going to analyze you (and your wardrobe) and come up with a tightly edited collection of fewer but better things. I won't limit you to a set number of items because the process will force you to only keep/buy what is essential – and that's all that matters.

We will follow the same 9-step process I used to create and maintain my own simple style. Plus, to assist you on your journey, I've created a complimentary companion guide you can access at **minimalism.co/style** so you can get the most out of the lessons.

There is one caveat. My goal is not to present you with the most original ideas about curating your wardrobe. My goal is to teach you how to simplify your style in as few words as possible. Because do you really need to sift through hundreds of pages of text to get the point? Of course not.

So this will be a brief book that helps you create a stylish but functional wardrobe that gives you confidence, in as little time as possible. Are you up for the challenge? Then let's get started!

Step 1: Match your wardrobe to your lifestyle

Life is as simple as these three questions: What do I want? Why do I want it? And, how will I achieve it? — Shannon L. Adler

I adore my wardrobe and it's a joy getting ready each day. I revel in the fact that I am so satisfied with the things I own, though I didn't always feel like this.

I used to stare at my closet for over 30 minutes stressing out about what to wear. I'd put on an outfit, immediately take it off, then try on something else and feel underwhelmed. Before I even made it out the door, I'd be frustrated and frazzled, then spend the rest of the day self-conscious about my look. It was a vicious cycle.

Sounds familiar?

Before you can perfect and streamline your style, you need to understand your lifestyle. If you have a lot of things in your closet that seem completely off, it is likely due to the fact that you are purchasing without first considering who you are, what you want to convey to the world, and the reality of your day-to-day.

An important step in the simple style process is mapping wardrobe to lifestyle, so what you wear is the best reflection of you. In addition to looking effortlessly stylish, I want you to feel comfortable and confident.

Your Challenge

Walk through the following three sets of questions which are important considerations for linking yourself to your style.

Self-reflection

These questions are all about having awareness, clarity, and focus.

- Who are you now and who do you want to be in the future?

- What do you (and do not) care about?

- On what do you tend to prioritize your resources (time, money, energy)?

Self-expression

After you finish the self-reflection exercise, it's time to think about self-expression and what you want to convey to the world with the following questions:

- What do you stand for and how does that drive the specific goals you want to achieve in the future?

- What special traits make you unique, important, relevant, and valuable to others?

- Summarize your personal aesthetic and the visible elements that allow you to express yourself.

Daily routine

Once you know who you are and how you express yourself – you now have to think about the reality of your daily life.

- Consider where your time goes during the week.

- What are the activities that matter most to you?

- Reflect on what a perfect day would look like for you.

If you don't understand and develop confidence in yourself, then how can you make clear and confident decisions about what to wear?

If you aren't sure how you want to present and express yourself to the world, won't lack of clarity show up in your style choices?

If you go through the day haphazardly with no daily routine, how can you dress comfortably and assertively to meet its demands?

The fundamentals of a simple style require using insights and cues from your lifestyle to inform and develop a clear sense of your personal style.

Step 2: Develop a distinct aesthetic

Create your own style ... let it be unique for yourself and yet identifiable for others
— Orson Welles

The ultimate benefit of a simple style is being able to have confidence in the way you look all the time. You can accomplish this by understanding your personal style and learning how to create outfits that reflect it.

In the last lesson we discussed the importance of self-awareness and self-expression, as well as understanding your daily routine. Now it's time to use those insights to cultivate a look that is quintessentially you.

Before I walk you through how to create your personal style, I want to share six reasons why this is such an important step in the process:

- You'll be able to get ready effortlessly because you know what works best for you.

- You'll develop a keen sense of quality and be drawn to well-made items.

- You'll be more motivated to properly care for your clothing and extend their life.

- You won't be swayed by trends because you'll have a unique "signature" style.

- You will no longer need external validation because of your strong sense of self.

- You'll be able to easily adapt your closet to different life stages (new job, new kid, etc.)

It's important to note that a simple style doesn't mean you can't let your natural aesthetic preferences shine through. I want to stress this point because I know a lot of people who are turned off by this concept because they automatically assume it requires you to have a minimalist aesthetic. This is absolutely false.

Your Challenge

It's time to get in touch with your own aesthetic, whatever that may be, so every single item of clothing you own is a piece you'll absolutely love.

Start with the basics

Here's a preliminary tip before you jump into assessing your own style. No matter your aesthetic (be it classic, boho, or edgy), you can benefit from having a selection of staples that represent the bulk of your wardrobe.

These staples (also known as basics) are foundational elements that can be worn frequently. Starting with them will almost completely eliminate the time you waste getting ready throughout the rest of the year.

Once you have your staples established, if you choose, you can embellish them with accessories or other more elaborate apparel pieces that help you create a signature look.

Gather inputs and inspiration

The following exercises will help you clearly visualize the types of things you love and feel confident wearing.

First, create a mood board using whatever method works for you (I recommend browsing online fashion magazines, blogs and Pinterest to find images). Save the outfits that you'd actually wear and jot down any common patterns or themes you notice.

Second, choose your style muses by determining 3-4 celebrities, influencers, public figures or people you know whose personal style you admire. Reflect on what attracts you to their style and make a list of the key attributes.

Now, move away from fashion and apparel and reflect on some of your favorite things and places. It can be a handbag you own or a museum you frequent. What about these things are you visually drawn to?

Create your personal style snapshot

In this final step, you will distill down all of your notes and insights into a succinct overview of your personal style.

Style — What are the types of looks and silhouettes that fit well with your aesthetic and lifestyle? List the words that best describe it (such as Preppy, Sporty, Urban, Bohemian, or Casual).

Colors — What palettes are you naturally drawn to? They don't necessarily have to be neutrals, but try to limit this list to 3-5 colors that work well together (making it easier to pull together outfits).

Fabrics — What materials do you feel most comfortable in and believe are best suited for your day-to-day? Consider natural fabrics such as cotton, linen, cashmere, and silk.

Outfits — Try to come up with your favorite looks based on your most common activities. For instance, what is your ideal outfit for work, weekend, and evenings out with friends or family?

Notes — Are there other considerations you need to be mindful of when it comes to your style? Jot down any important notes that haven't already been captured.

Step 3: Evaluate what should stay or go

*Edit your life frequently and ruthlessly.
It's your masterpiece after all.*
— Nathan W. Morris

Now that you know your personal style, it's time to make changes to your wardrobe to reflect it. This is where we get into the nitty gritty of the book because you will start to make direct edits to your closet.

There are three steps to evaluating and editing your wardrobe:

- Reviewing your personal style

- Removing unwanted items

- Reassessing what you have vs. need

Your Challenge

Walk through the following exercises to edit your closet according to your lifestyle and aesthetic.

Review your personal style

Reflect on your lifestyle and your personal aesthetic as a refresher for this lesson.

Go through your closet and pull out anything that doesn't immediately feel relevant, useful or meaningful.

Remove unwanted items

Sort your pile according to things you will throw away vs. give away. If you are hesitant to get rid of an item, take note of it and keep it in your closet for another month or two. If you don't wear it after that time, then remove it. If you choose to hold onto an item for sentimental vs. functional reasons, that's ok so long as it doesn't contribute to clutter in your closet.

Reassess what you have vs. need

Take inventory of what's left and take note of any items that you need to add or replace. We'll address this list in the next lesson.

Step 4: Create a shopping checklist

In character, in manner, in style, in all things, the supreme excellence is simplicity. — Henry Wadsworth Longfellow

Now that you've completed the closet evaluation, it's time to start finalizing your wardrobe. You'll do this by developing a nifty checklist and referencing it to figure out what you have and what you need.

Your Challenge

The easiest way to do this is to review the list of outfits organized by lifestyle that you created in Step 3. Break the outfits down into categories, such as:

- Tops

- Bottoms

- Shoes

- Outwear

- Accessories

Then compare this list to what you already have in your closet (what you've decided to keep after Step 4). Whatever is missing should be added to your shopping list.

Once you've finalized the list, try to order the items by importance, just in case you aren't able to purchase everything at one time. You want to get the most important pieces first — namely staples and any other items that show up repeatedly in multiple outfits.

Step 5: Budget for any wardrobe needs

Never use the word "cheap". Today everybody can look chic in inexpensive clothes. There is good clothing design on every level today. You can be the chicest thing in the world in a T-shirt and jeans ... it's up to you. — Karl Lagerfeld

Before you rush off to shop, I want to address your budget, as it's important that you stay within your financial means. The budgeting challenge is a simple exercise to ensure you don't go broke. It makes no sense getting into debt trying to simplify your style!

These days you don't need a big budget to dress well. There are a plethora of brands available across different price points (we'll get into them in the next lesson). Because of the options, most people enjoy dressing "high and low" despite their socio-economic status. So don't be tempted to stretch your budget to accommodate a shopping spree.

Your Challenge

Calculate your total monthly income from wages, investments, and any other forms of cash inflows. Be sure to adjust the amount for taxes to get an estimated net income figure.

Calculate your total monthly expenses. This should include Home, Transportation, Insurance, Food, Savings, and other core living expenses.

Deduct your total expenses from your total income to get a "disposable" or discretionary income figure. This is what you have available for spending after your essential needs are met.

Determine how much of your discretionary funds you feel comfortable allocating to your wardrobe monthly vs. other things or experiences. That amount is what you have available to purchase the items on your shopping list.

Depending on your budget, you may not be able to get everything on your shopping list at one time. So select the most essential items for this month and plan to get the rest in subsequent months.

Step 6: Determine a set of "go-to" brands

I have the simplest tastes. I am only satisfied with the best. — Oscar Wilde

I am a strong advocate of having a go-to set of brands that you can depend on for your simple style. This lesson will discuss how to discover those brands and provide recommendations on where to start.

As a former fashion marketing executive, I've noticed a shift in how our generation perceives the role of fashion brands and designers. More and more, the fashion brand or designer is expected to tackle the complexities around utility (e.g. fit and fabrication) while leaving the more nebulous interpretation of beauty (e.g. styling) to the wearer of the garment.

To be clear, customers are starting to prefer defining their own style. Instead of allowing their sense of self, worth and style to be manipulated by marketing jargon, they want brands to focus on perfecting the quality of the goods they offer.

Now that you know what you need to purchase and how much you can afford to spend, I want to help you choose brands that prioritize quality to help maximize the bang for your buck.

Your Challenge

The main benefit of having a go-to list of brands is that you'll know without a doubt what works for your style, your body type, and your budget. There are five primary considerations for creating your go-to brand list:

Quality

When choosing a brand, the first element to investigate is quality, as I mentioned earlier. Read the brand's website and seek quality assurance cues such as an overview of their fabrication and manufacturing techniques, a discussion on where their items are made, and whether they have a rich heritage or longstanding tradition in their category.

A brand that cares about quality will want to showcase it via beautiful lifestyle and product images, behind the scenes snapshots of their showroom and factories, interesting vignettes about how their fabric is sourced, their branding and packaging, etc. Also, read any reviews you can find to get feedback from fellow customers.

Fit

Not all brands conform to the same sizing standards, so measure yourself or go to a local tailor to get your body measurements (in inches or centimeters) before you go brand hunting.

If you are shopping in-store, then try on everything before buying if you aren't familiar with how a brand fits you. When shopping online, navigate to the size guide (usually on the product pages or in the FAQs) to see how your measurements translate.

Many brands are also starting to enhance the buying experience with richer fit descriptions, better product images and video (so you can see how the item falls on the body), and tech solutions which use data to help customers find the perfect size.

Price

Believe it or not, "you get what you pay for" is not always true. As a former fashion marketing executive, I can tell you truthfully that price does not always translate to quality. Nevertheless, it is useful to tier brands by price point to get a sense of where you need to shop based on your budget.

- Couture ($2000)

- Luxury ($500)

- Affordable Luxury ($225)

- Premium ($85)

- Fast Fashion ($50)

- Budget ($10)

The figures in parentheses are back of envelope averages for the price of a women's dress at full retail. I recognize there may be different interpretations of this, and many brands have offerings in multiple tiers, but this should do for a rough assessment.

I personally believe Premium and Affordable Luxury brands offer the best cost-to-value and, at times, the quality differentiation between the two is hard to detect. So if you are forced to opt for a lower priced item, it won't necessarily mean a major decrease in quality.

Some Fast Fashion brands can hold up quite well, especially if they offer special edition collections that tend to be better crafted. The overall experience and quality of goods at Budget brands are likely too poor to bother with. Nevertheless, if financial restraints force you to shop at these stores, always choose basics over trendy pieces and put more effort into caring for the items so they don't fall apart.

Once you establish your price range and the categories you fall into, it'll take a bit of trial and error with fit and quality to nail your go-to list.

Service

Because there is so much competition in the retail industry and a plethora of options, I have a zero tolerance personal policy for bad service. There is no reason to patronize a brand that doesn't exhibit A+ customer service.

The most important things to look for as it pertains to service are usually found in the FAQs. Search for things like a free and easy return policy, fast and affordable shipping, warranty for defective goods and an effortless way to contact the brand.

Mission

Connecting with a brand on a higher level can help you narrow your list. Take some time to learn about their corporate policies, company culture, and reputation in the press, and see if they resonate with any of your personal ideals.

Now that you know what to look for in a brand, here's how to conduct research in order to craft your list:

Closet

Look at what you already own. Go to your closet, pull out 3-5 pieces that you absolutely love wearing, and jot down the brand names. Add these brands to your consideration list and use them as a reference for the type of aesthetic that you are drawn to and the price point that you fall within.

Online

Pinterest is an excellent way to conduct brand research because of its strong visuals and popularity with lifestyle categories like fashion. Because it is a visual search engine, it is more efficient for your brand research than searching Google.

Perform 3-4 word, highly descriptive searches (such as "minimal chic style") and use the automatic suggestion boxes at the top of the feed to dive deeper. Then just scroll through looking for beautiful images and following the links to any outfits that resonate.

Referrals

As I mentioned, friends, bloggers, and even celebrities can be great sources of ideas. The key is that their recommendations need to be properly vetted against the five elements outlined above.

Think about any individuals you know (or know of) whose style is a close reflection of what you are trying to accomplish with your own wardrobe. Either reach out to them (if they are someone you can directly contact) or visit their social media channels and see if they promote any brands in particular. Gather the names and add them to your consideration list.

Step 7: Shop without impulse purchasing

Women usually love what they buy, yet hate two-thirds of what is in their closets. — Mignon McLaughlin

Finally, it's time to shop, and this lesson will make your excursion extremely efficient. It's been my experience from working with clients on personal branding and self-image that both genders experience issues from not knowing how to shop effectively.

Now that you have your list of items, list of brands, and budget set, you have everything you need to go out and refresh your wardrobe. But I want you to be smart about this. You didn't come this far only to end up (once again) with a bunch of stuff you don't need.

Your Challenge

Let's get organized in order to avoid the impulse shopping trap. You'll use the following checks and balances to help avoid unnecessary purchases.

Schedule your shopping excursion

With the exception of groceries, general household items, and the occasional unexpected or special situation that calls for a sporadic new purchase, I personally schedule major shopping initiatives at the beginning of each quarter (four times a year corresponding with seasonal changes).

I refer to my list and then go through the process of eliminating things I don't really want or need, determining new things I want or need, and prioritizing based on my budget. I then buy solely what ends up left on the list.

When you schedule your shopping excursions they become important events that you can thoughtfully prepare for vs. a bunch of random one-off impulse buys.

Bring your list with you

Impulse purchases are driven by impulse emotions. For instance, you scroll through Instagram, see something nice, navigate to the website, and end up being sucked into the trap.

Always add an item to your shopping list and let it sit on the list for a while before you decide to purchase it. This will not only give you time to consider whether you really need it, but also allow you to compare its importance to other items on your list.

Even better is to create a master list of essential items that you've thought about and know work best for your style and life. Then the only time you need to shop is when you have to replace an item that's on this list.

Stay true to your style

You've gone through the process of understanding your aesthetic and having go-to brands that work well with your style. Try to respect your unique aesthetic when shopping instead of falling prey to marketing tactics that lure you into buying something that's not right for you.

I don't want to encourage you to be close-minded. Experimentation and exploration is a very important part of self-expression and establishing and evolving your personal sense of style. The key here is that you recognize when an item is too far off from your style, and have the discipline to say no despite how lovely it may be.

Step 8: Increase the longevity of your clothing

Mankind has built oh so many perfect things! — Pablo Neruda

The fewer items you have the better they should be cared for, and in this lesson I want to share tips on how to extend the longevity of your wardrobe. Before getting into those tips, however, I want to throw out one word: gratitude.

Take a moment and consider how far you've come since you started this book. Then I want you to express gratitude — just be thankful for the fact that you now have a beautiful and functional wardrobe that will give you the confidence to address the demands of the day.

Your Challenge

When you are thankful for the things you have, you are more likely to respect and properly care for them. Now that you've curated your perfect closet, use these simple fabric care tips to be mindful of the upkeep of your items and extend their longevity.

You may have your own special tricks for caring for your wardrobe, but here's a simple and handy guide with general rules of thumb for properly maintaining items.

I strongly recommend natural materials because they are environmentally friendly and don't contain chemicals that irritate the skin, so this guide focuses on organic fabrics.

Cashmere

- Cold hand wash

- Air dry flat on towel

- Store folded

Cotton

- Wash warm on normal cycle

- Bleach whites if needed

- Tumble dry and iron okay

- Can be folded or hung

Denim

- Cold delicate wash (sparingly)

- Turn inside out in wash

- Air dry flat

- Store folded

Leather

- Treat with protector before wearing

- Spot wipe with damp cloth

- Hang jackets on sturdy wood hanger

- Avoid rain and wet conditions

Linen

- Warm delicate wash

- Air dry flat or on rack

- Iron on wrong side (linen setting)

- Hang in closet

Silk

- Dry clean or cool hand wash

- Low heat iron on silk setting

- Use mesh bag for intimates

- Hang clothing, fold intimates

Wool

- Delicate wash sweaters (wool cycle)

- Air dry sweaters flat on towel

- Dry clean wool coats (before storing)

- Hang coats on sturdy wood hangers

- Fold all others

General Tips

Treat your items with a sense of respect i.e. do not ever throw your clothing on the floor, step on them, or leave them balled up in the corner of the room for days on end.

Wash intimates, swimwear, and workout gear after wearing. Everything else you can typically wear about 3-4 times before washing, except for coats which you can dry-clean at the end of the season.

When washing, use gentle chemical-free detergents, wash with like colors (and fabrics if possible), and if ever in doubt, follow the manufacturer's cleaning instructions. Though I mention ironing, I actually prefer a steamer as it doesn't come into direct contact with the material.

Always clean items before placing in seasonal storage and use breathable, well-sealed, fabric storage bags. Cedar chips will keep moths away.

Step 9: Maintain your commitment to a simple style

We must always change, renew, rejuvenate ourselves; otherwise, we harden. — Johann Wolfgang von Goethe

You are almost at the finish line. Congratulations! I'll close out the book by discussing how you can maintain and stay committed to your newly created simple style over time. After all this work we wouldn't want you to revert back to a closet full of stuff you don't adore!

My personal method and recommendation is to refresh on a quarterly basis. All you need to do is schedule time in your calendar to repeat lessons 4-8:

- Re-evaluate your closet — it should be much easier next time

- Make your shopping list — it should be much shorter next time

- Review your budget — and stay within your means

- Determine your brands — start with your go-to list

- Schedule your shopping excursion and voila!

Your Challenge

Schedule time on a monthly or quarterly basis to refresh your closet by quickly reviewing the step-by-step lessons in this book. Then download the companion guide at <u>minimalism.co/style</u> which allows you to pull together all of your thoughts into one place.

Resources

I'm thrilled you've made it through the entire Style Challenge! This brief book was designed to be a lightweight style guide. Instead of overwhelming you with templates, worksheets and lengthy instructions my goal was to get straight to the point so you can curate your personal style sooner than later.

However even though this was intended to be a short guide there is still quite a bit of material covered. It may take time to process the information and develop a personal plan for integrating the recommendations into your closet.

Don't feel discouraged if you find you need more time and support converting to a simple style. Although the changes are small, they are significant. That's because you aren't just updating your wardrobe or refreshing your closet — you are learning how to be more intentional with your time, energy, and money.

To assist you on your style journey I've developed a companion guide that you can download at minimalism.co/style to help you make the most of the book.

Books

I'm sure it's safe to assume that simplifying your style is only one of many ways in which you aim to commit to personal growth. If you've picked up this book then you are likely also motivated to develop other areas of your life as well, be it wellness, finances, career or relationships.

Well, you are in luck. It's both my purpose and my pleasure to present you with more simple strategies for streamlining life — based on years of observing, researching and synthesizing what's essential for a well-lived lifestyle.

I'm no philosopher but I am a personal growth and business coach, and I have to tackle big life themes on a daily basis — for myself and the thousands of clients I serve through my work.

If you'd like to continue improving yourself, I invite you to explore the other books in the Streamline Your Life series at **minimalism.co/books** which include:

The Minimalism Challenge: 52 small changes and good habits that will simplify your life each week of the year

The Sleep Challenge: 14 simple sleep solutions to get more and better sleep in only 14 nights

The Self-Care Challenge: simplify your well-being with this 12-step healthy living framework

Author

A. Edmond is a personal growth coach, business and brand strategist, creative entrepreneur and digital influencer. Previously, she was a marketing executive in the fashion and luxury space and, before that, a financial analyst.

She's built a following of over 100,000 readers, hundreds of individual coaching clients and a roster of a dozen iconic and Fortune 500 brands using her intuitive yet strategic approach to personal and business growth. In total her work has reached over 1 million like-minded individuals.

With over a decade of personal and professional development experience, A. Edmond has a knack for leveraging her unique blend of creative and analytical skills to help others improve their lives and develop their life's work.

A. Edmond works independently and currently focuses most of her efforts on coaching and developing books and courses for fellow independent spirits — creative entrepreneurs who desire freedom, fulfillment and financial success.

A. Edmond received her MBA from the Stanford Graduate School of Business. Prior to being an entrepreneur and coach she worked with and advised iconic brands such as Disney, JPMorganChase, Ralph Lauren, eBay, Procter & Gamble, and many more.